Having your first baby

by

Sister Jean Fielding, SRN

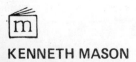

KENNETH MASON

Contents

Introduction

If you are having your first baby this is one year in your life that you will remember specially. Having a baby can be a delight-ful and satisfying experience, provided you are able to keep in good health, and allay certain natural enxieties. By learning a little about your body and the organs involved in pregnancy and what happens to them during the waiting months, you will better understand how to keep happy and relaxed.

This book gives a simple account of the changes which take place in your mind and body during pregnancy and explains how you can cope with them and enjoy them.

To enable you to keep well during pregnancy it is advisable to seek medical advice immediately you consider you are preg-nant. Regular visits to your doctor or ante-natal clinic are essen-tial as a safeguard against any of the complications of pregnancy. Ante-natal care and teaching are invaluable because they help you to develop a peaceful mind and fit body so that you ap-proach the birth of your baby with cheerful confidence.

Your husband has his part to play and should fully under-stand the processes involved in pregnancy so that he can provide support and help when you require them. If possible, encourage him to attend an ante-natal class arranged for fathers.

The experiences you will have during labour are often influ-enced by your childhood, your education about sex and child-hood and your marriage relationship.

Fortunately most of the preconceived fears and misunder-standings about pregnancy and childbirth can be dispelled if you accept the aids of modern science and follow your doctor's advice.

This book is aimed at helping you to look forward to nine happy months and to producing a healthy baby. If you practise simple exercises regularly throughout pregnancy they will help you to keep fit and look better. Ideally these should be learned under the supervision of an expert but if there is no ante-natal class in your district, follow the exercises and instruction about breathing and relaxation techniques included in this book. The importance of eating a well-balanced diet and of avoiding an excessive weight gain is also stressed.

If you are well-adjusted during pregnancy you should find labour an exhilarating experience. Scientific advances in recent years have helped to make childbirth safer than ever before. The excellent facilities available through the Health Service do everything possible to ensure a good pregnancy, a safe and enjoyable labour and a successful start to your baby's life.

You will obtain the best obstetric attention in the world from your obstetrician, doctors and midwives for a greater understanding of the needs of a pregnant woman — physical, mental and emotional — exists today.

1 Are you pregnant?

The first indication of a possible pregnancy is often an occasional feeling of dizziness with bouts of nausea and morning sickness. If you are pregnant you may notice tingling of the breasts and the need to pass urine more frequently due to a slightly enlarged uterus pressing on the bladder. When you have missed a period you will be anxious to have your pregnancy confirmed, although sometimes a breakdown in the menstrual cycle may be caused by ill-health, environmental changes, anxiety, wishful thinking or the approach of the menopause.

As you are known to your doctor he is the person you should consult for confirmation of your pregnancy. If you do not wish to wait until you have missed two periods, delay your visit until a fortnight after your period was due. The most certain way of establishing a diagnosis is by means of a pregnancy test which will be positive about 12 days after the first day of the missed period if you have conceived.

Your doctor will advise you about the ante-natal clinic service. Although he may run his own, most doctors refer patients to local ante-natal clinics which are well-equipped.

Comparatively few babies are born at home now and your doctor will want you to have your first baby in hospital. He will refer you to the nearest maternity hospital where in due course you can chat to the midwife. It is reassuring to see inside the hospital for you will be encouraged to see how happy the women are after having delivered their offspring only a few hours earlier.

You may feel shy or embarrassed when you visit your doctor on this first occasion but he is going to be your good friend during the months ahead and will soon dispel your fears. Do not hesitate to ask him about any problems which have been worrying you and he will try to solve them.

If you wish your husband to be present during labour mention this to your doctor to enable him to refer you to a hospital or nursing home where husbands are allowed to attend the birth. If you are afraid of having a painful labour and have read about the advantages of epidural analgesia discuss this with your doctor. He will explain that although the pain-killing drugs which are injected into the lower back are most effective they are not suitable for all women. Also, they require a great deal of valuable medical time. Admittedly, American women have been given epidurals for years but they pay their gynaecologists exorbitant fees for the privilege.

When you visit your doctor take an early morning specimen of urine although he may prefer to test a 'mid-stream' specimen. To obtain this, you will be asked to pass some urine at the surgery and then collect a small amount in a sterile container. Much the most reliable confirmation of pregnancy is a chemical test on your urine. There are a number of these tests which can detect hormones secreted by the developing foetus and its placenta. By examining this urine your doctor can discover if you have any infection of the urinary tract which might cause kidney disease during pregnancy.

Your urine will be tested for protein for its presence might indicate the possibility of pre-eclampsia occurring later in pregnancy. This condition is specific to pregnancy and the cause is still unknown despite a considerable amount of research. In eclampsia a raised blood pressure results in protein being shed from the kidneys and appearing in the urine. Swelling of the feet, ankles or hands occurs and usually an excessive weight gain is noted.

One important aspect of the care of a pregnant woman in the ante-natal clinic is always directed towards the prevention of pre-eclampsia (toxaemia). Routine urine tests are performed at every ante-natal visit during pregnancy to detect the presence of protein and sugar. When sugar is discovered, or if a woman is a known diabetic, she must receive regular medical supervision throughout pregnancy as a very high blood sugar or an overdose of insulin can prove harmful to the foetus just as it can to the pregnant woman herself.

Your doctor will check your weight and height, listen to your heart with a stethoscope and check your blood pressure. This is an essential procedure during ante-natal visits as a raised blood pressure may lead to pre-eclampsia or the more severe condition of eclampsia. If detected early and treated correctly this condition will not affect mother or child.

Your doctor will ask you several routine questions including: 'What illnesses and operations have you had?' He wants this information in case any condition needs treatment to prevent it affecting the course of your pregnancy. If you have had any miscarriages or abortions it is essential for you to give full details to the doctor so that he can anticipate complications.

One early question will be: 'When was your last period and how often do you have a period?' When doctor knows how many days or weeks have passed since your missed period, the date of the first day of your last period and the normal length of your menstrual cycle he can calculate approximately the date on which your baby is likely to be born.

A normal pregnancy lasts for 40 weeks. Your baby's birthdate is found by adding seven days and nine calendar months to the first day of the last normal period eg first day of last period — Jan 1, 1979, expected date of delivery — Sept 8, 1979.

You will be asked: 'Do you have any tingling of the breasts and does your brassiere feel tight?' The breasts start to enlarge early in pregnancy and a feeling of fullness may be experienced as early as the third week. Doctor will examine the breasts to see if the nipples have gone darker in colour and look more prominent and if the pigmented areas around them have become larger. He may ask if some veins are more noticeable recently. If you intend to breastfeed your baby your doctor may suggest certain manipulations which you can do during pregnancy to encourage milk production and make the establishment of breastfeeding easier. If your nipples are small or inverted, he may advise you to wear 'Woolwich Breast Shields' inside your bra regularly from the fourth month to draw out the nipples and relieve pressure on them.

Your doctor will ask: 'Have you any varicose veins?' for these tend to become more pronounced during pregnancy owing to increased pressure from the enlarging uterus. If necessary he will advise you to wear support tights and to rest your legs in an elevated position whenever possible.

Doctor enquires: 'Are your clothes feeling tighter round the waist?' because he knows that the abdomen sometimes starts to swell even before the breasts.

Frequency in passing urine is almost universal during early pregnancy so you will be asked: 'Do you have to pass water at night and do you go more often during the day?'

'Have you gone off any foods or do you feel off food early in the morning?' Doctor knows that lack of appetite is common at this time. He will prove sympathetic if you cannot enjoy food because of morning sickness and may suggest ways to control the nausea or vomiting.

When your doctor asks: 'Have you any vaginal discharge?,' he does not imply that you necessarily have some infection. Extra moisture appears in the vagina during pregnancy and may cause a slight discharge which is quite normal.

You will be asked to undress and lie on a couch where doctor will examine you internally by passing a small instrument into the vagina. This simple examination takes only a minute or two and causes the minimum of discomfort if you try to relax. Doctor assesses the size of the birth canal and can see if the vagina has become a mauvish colour as this is an early indication of pregnancy. After inspecting the cervix (neck of the uterus) for a similar colour change, he may take a 'Pap smear' test. Besides providing valuable information about any risk of cancer in the years ahead the test shows gland changes which are important for the maintenance of pregnancy. It also reveals if any mild infections are present which can be treated before the baby is born.

Several important tests will be carried out on a sample of blood which doctor will take from a vein in your arm. This procedure is not painful and the information obtained is most valuable.

It is vital for you to feel able to ask your doctor for accurate information at all times during your pregnancy. He will gladly advise you about suitable diet, exercise or coping with minor troubles encountered during pregnancy. He will tell you to report to him any unexpected pain, vaginal bleeding, exceptional tiredness or weight gain, swelling of the ankles or the development of varicose veins or piles.

2 Your baby's development

Although the embryo is very tiny during the first month of pregnancy, it begins developing into a human infant before it is more than 1.5 cm (½ in) in length. An elementary head starts forming about the third week, then the brain and spinal cord begin to develop while early signs of muscle formation occur. Gradually on the sides of the embryo swellings appear which are limb 'buds' and will later become arms. The legs follow a few days later. The kidneys, liver and digestive system begin to develop although at four weeks the embryo bears no resemblance to a baby.

By eight weeks the embryo is 2.5 cm (1 in) long and looks

more like a human. The head is large compared to the body and the external ears are forming. The limb buds are now arms and legs, the eyelids now cover the eyes and all the main organs of the body have formed. The heart is beating, blood circulates through its vessels, the stomach is active and the kidneys are starting to function.

At 12 weeks the uterus is rising out of the pelvis. The foetus (young one) is 9 cm (3½ in) long. The head is still over-large, nails have appeared on fingers and toes and the external genitals are appearing. Tiny movements of the arms and legs occur, and the foetus can swallow and pass urine.

The uterus is reaching halfway to the umbilicus by the 16th week and is beginning to make a bulge. The foetus measures 18 cm (7 in) in length and weighs 100 g (4 oz). The body is bright red because blood vessels show through the transparent skin. Its heart beats strongly, muscles are becoming active and the sex can be distinguished. Now the weight of the placenta and foetus are about equal.

By 20 weeks the foetus is distinctly human in appearance and has 'quickened'. It is about 25 cm (10 in) long and weighs about 300 g (11 oz). The skin has thickened and is completely covered with downy hair (lanugo). Hair is appearing on its head and eyebrows have developed but the eyelids are still closed.

Around 24 weeks the foetus measures 32 cm (13 in) and weighs 650 g (1 lb 7 oz). The skin is less red, though still covered with lanugo and is wrinkled. Its eyelids are separated now and the head is still comparatively large.

Your baby's heart can be heard distinctly by the doctor at 28 weeks. The foetus is 38 cm (15 in) long and weighs 1000 g (2 lb 2 oz). Its body is thin, the reddish skin is covered with a creamy substance called *vernix caseosa*. It can open its eyes, move around vigorously in the uterus and is able to breathe and cry weakly. If born now, it may survive.

At 32 weeks the foetus measures 43 cm (17 in) long and weighs 1,800 g (4 lb). Some fat is being deposited under the skin. The bones of the head are soft and flexible. The lungs have developed and can now support life if necessary.

By 36 weeks the foetus reaches up to the rib-cage. It is 46 cm (18½ in) long and 2,500 g (5½ lb) in weight. The foetus has filled out as more fat has been deposited beneath the skin. The face is round and is no longer wrinkled. Finger nails reach to the tips of the fingers.

When the pregnancy reaches full term at 40 weeks the baby is 3,300 g (7 lb 4 oz). A boy will be about 100 g (3 oz) heavier than a girl. Baby's skin is smooth and the lanugo has disappeared except over the shoulders. The skin is still covered with the *vernix caseosa* and the head is covered with hair in varying amounts. The head now measures about one quarter of the body's length. Although the eyes are open they are usually a dull slate colour, but the permanent colour will appear later. The baby is now 8 million times heavier than the original fertilized cell.

3 Diet really does matter

The old wives' tale which suggests 'A pregnant woman should eat enough for two' is dangerous advice as overeating leads to overweight with its resulting problems. You do not require a special diet during pregnancy but you do need well-balanced meals containing a good supply of proteins, mineral salts and vitamins.

Our average diet today consists largely of refined, prepared, processed, over-cooked, tinned and devitalized foods. Many natural minerals and vitamins are destroyed during the preserving and manufacture of foods.

During pregnancy which is a period of great physiological activity your body has an increased need for mineral salts and vitamins. If your diet is deficient in these elements you may feel weary, lack enthusiasm for living, suffer from nausea, decaying teeth or falling hair, or lose your good looks. Unless you improve your diet you may have a painful labour while your baby may be less healthy than could have been expected.

Rules for choosing your foods

1   Select foods of the best nutritional quality throughout your pregnancy to give your baby the finest possible start in life.
2   Fruits and vegetables should form about two-thirds of your diet.
3   Include a wide variety of protein foods.
4   Eat as much food as possible raw. Cooking destroys many

10

important vitamins, minerals and trace elements.
5   Wholegrain cereals and natural sugars are best.
6   Eat 'whole' natural foods which are health-giving.
7   Dairy produce is important.
8   When possible, buy organically grown food.

Adequate good protein

Protein is the food for building muscles and other tissues, so a fair amount is essential for a successful pregnancy. Eat lean meat if you enjoy it though a good vegetarian dietary in which proteins are derived from milk, yoghourt, eggs, cheese, nuts, 100 per cent wholewheat bread and pulse foods (peas, beans, lentils, soya flour) is perfect for expectant mothers. Vegetable proteins do not give the kidneys so much work to do as meat and meat products.

Dairy produce and other fats

You require comparatively little actual fat because some is present in protein foods, such as meat, cheese, eggs and milk. It is best to avoid cream and fat meat especially if you gain weight easily. If you find difficulty in digesting fats, buy extra lean meats and fish and grill them. Eat curd cheese instead of hard cheeses. Use a vegetable oil for cooking protein foods and use just sufficient butter to make toast or bread palatable.

Milk, cheese, eggs and yoghourt are valuable because of their high calcium content. If you are not fond of milk, take extra yoghourt, preferably goat's milk or natural yoghourt. Eggs are a splendid source of protein and mineral salts, particularly iron and phosphorus and contain more calcium, vitamins A, D and B and riboflavin than beef.

Vitamins and minerals

Most of our foods contain mineral salts and vitamins which are vital food factors. During pregnancy you need a constant supply of all the different mineral salts or the foetus will take his requirements from your body.

Most doctors give tablets containing iron and folic acid, a vitamin of the B group because a deficiency of them may cause anaemia. As extra calcium is necessary, you must either drink extra milk, eat more cheese or take calcium tablets three times daily.

Carbohydrate foods

Recent research has proved that a diet high in carbohydrates will increase your weight more than a high-calorie diet consisting mainly of proteins and fats. Fortunately our bodies need few sugars and starches. Carbohydrates provide an instant source of energy but any excess is converted into fat and deposited in the body.

Fruits and vegetables

The two-thirds of your diet made up of fruit and vegetables includes potatoes, dried fruit, nuts and pulse foods (peas, beans and lentils). Fresh fruits are ideal for you because of their high content of minerals and vitamins and because they are easily digested even when morning sickness is present. Take acid fruits such as plums, strawberries and grapefruit with discretion but oranges suit most pregnant women.

Besides supplying minerals and vitamins, vegetables provide bulk and roughage which assist in the proper elimination of waste products and most of them are easily digested.

Nuts are nutritious and easily digested when milled. Lentils provide an excellent source of natural iron.

Although bottled fruits and tinned fruits and vegetables give variety and are useful for occasional meals, do not allow them to take the place of fresh fruits and vegetables regularly.

If you are gaining weight too quickly, start each meal with raw fruit to curb your appetite for more fattening foods.

Wholegrain cereals

Wholewheat bread made from 100 per cent flour will provide you with valuable protein, iron, calcium, phosphorus, magnesium and various trace elements, the essential vitamin B complex, vitamin E and essential unsaturated fatty acids.

You need these for creating a perfect baby. If you cannot buy 100 per cent wholewheat bread, it is easy to make at home. A recent survey proved that if you eat wholewheat bread during pregnancy it will help your baby to have sound teeth. Include whole rice, rye and oatmeal in your diet occasionally.

Natural sugars

When you require a sweetener, choose nature's own sugar, honey. Buy pure honey, not blended. Use Barbados sugar and black treacle in moderation for they retain valuable nutrients which are removed during the refining of white sugar. Sweet dried fruits — raisins, dates and figs — are sources of natural sugar which are ideal for you as they are not over-concentrated and provide nutrients as well as sugar.

Value of raw foods

Raw food is particularly beneficial, especially raw fruits and vegetables since even the most careful cooking destroys some of their minerals and vitamins. Ideally, you should enjoy a salad daily but if you cannot tolerate raw vegetables at times, drink freshly pressed fruit and vegetable juices instead.

Try to take some of your milk as fresh milk and not heated up as coffee or cocoa. Another excellent raw food is muesli which is a perfect breakfast dish.

Muesli recipe

Stir together one tablespoon of medium oatmeal or oat-flakes and three tablespoons of water. Leave to soak overnight, then add lemon juice to taste, a grated unpeeled apple, raisins, nuts, honey and a little top milk. Add wheatgerm if desired or any fruit in season.

Eat whole foods for health

Eat your apple unpeeled or you will miss the roughage value of the skin and the nutrients such as magnesium, phosphorus and silicin which are concentrated just below the skin. Cook potatoes in their skins to conserve all the nutrients. When you peel a potato, besides losing the nutrients under the skin, you lose more in the cooking water. Baked potatoes can often be eaten comfortably when morning sickness is troublesome.

A sensible eating routine

To avoid tummy upsets or sickness and to obtain the full nourishment from food during pregnancy:

1 Eat your meals dry and drink fluids between them and at least half-an-hour before the next meal and two hours after the previous one.
2 Chew all your food thoroughly and eat slowly.
3 Try to avoid rushing a meal and eat it with enjoyment — if you are tense or overtired, try to relax before eating your food.
4 Avoid all highly spiced foods, fried and twice cooked foods, fancy cakes, pastries and salt.
5 Meat is not essential provided you eat other protein foods.
6 If you practise regular deep breathing this helps with the proper digestion and assimilation of the food eaten.
7 Always have one pint of milk daily and plenty of pure water, and fresh fruit and vegetable juices. Avoid fruit squashes which have a high white sugar content.
8 Avoid alcohol, especially spirits, although an occasional glass of dry sherry or wine with a meal is harmless. If your appetite is poor, a little wine may stimulate it and enable you to enjoy your food.
9 Try to avoid eating snacks between meals. A drink of milk or Marmite is satisfying but if really hungry, chew an apple, raw carrot or some celery.
10 Restrict salt as much as possible except in cooking. If you must use salt buy iodised table salt or sea salt from a health food store (salt encourages the retention of fluids in the body tissues).

4 Regular exercises are helpful

Although ideally every pregnant woman would benefit from attending classes held at ante-natal clinics, many cannot join a group because they are working full-time, or because there is no ante-natal class within a reasonable travelling distance.

By practising ante-natal exercises daily from the fourth month of pregnancy, a woman helps to keep herself in good health, maintain a comfortable posture, helps to make her labour easier and ensures that her figure will return to normal fairly quickly after delivery. Learning to breathe and relax properly can definitely make labour easier and quicker, as the earlier pioneers, Dr Grantley Dick Reade and Dr Pierre Lamaze preached for years.

Simple exercises before and after the birth of your baby will help you to keep well and look better. During pregnancy they will help to prevent overstretching of the muscles of the abdomen and those surrounding the birth canal.

You must learn how to balance your altering weight and to minimise strain which can result in chronic backache. All movements are helpful as they stimulate the circulation of your blood even by means of breathing exercises and simple foot and leg exercises.

A daily exercise routine

Practise these exercises regularly, preferably during the morning before you become tired. If you are a working wife, do them before your bedtime bath.

Lie on your back with knees bent and feet resting flat on the floor. Breathe in deeply, then exhale slowly. Repeat three times. This exercise encourages you to use your lungs fully and stimulates your blood circulation.

Do this between exercises and when the session is completed.

1   Sit on a bed or sofa with your back supported and your legs stretched straight out and slightly apart. Bend your ankles forwards as far as possible, then backwards, six times.
    Next, roll your feet in circles inwards, then outwards, six times. These exercises help to prevent you grumbling: 'My feet are so tired.'

2   Lie on your back with knees bent. Tighten up your buttock muscles and pull in your tummy hard. Check that there is no hollow under your back. Repeat six times. Learn to practise this movement in any position. It helps to keep your pelvic muscles in good condition and to prevent a sagging abdomen after baby's birth.

3   Keep in the same position and pull in your vaginal muscles. Relax and repeat six times. This exercise strengthens the muscles which support the uterus. Practise it often in any position as it will prevent the vaginal walls from becoming over-stretched during the birth.

4   Lie on your back with hands by your sides. Raise your right leg upwards then lower it slowly. Repeat six times with both legs. Relax, then perform twenty cycling 'kicks' using both legs. These movements help to prevent swollen ankles and

15

varicose veins as they improve the circulation in the legs.

5 Breathing exercises

Lie on back with a small pillow under the head. Keep knees bent and feet flat on the floor.

a Breathe in deeply and slowly, making tummy rise and fall. Repeat six times.

b Breathe with chest only, as deeply as possible for six times.

c Draw in a deep breath, hold it then allow the air to escape slowly. Repeat six times.

d Open your mouth and pant gently, taking shallow breaths. Repeat twelve times.

6 Breast-toner

Fold arms while sitting on a hard-backed chair. Grasp opposite fore-arms near elbows with each hand. Grip tightly then try to push the skin towards the elbows in short jerks. You should feel a pull in your breasts. Repeat at least ten times daily.

7 Donkey exercise

Kneel down, then place hands on floor, keeping your back parallel with the floor. Contract your tummy and arch your back gently. Relax. Repeat six times. (If any floor-polishing has to be done, this proves an excellent exercise, too.)

8 Leg-bending

Place feet apart, turned slightly outwards, and squat down, keeping arms forwards and heels on the ground. Now, rise up again. If necessary, place your hands on edge of the bath or bed for support. Repeat ten times daily, as this stretches the tissues and mobilises the joints ready for the actual birth. Use this position when possible if doing jobs like polishing furniture, or cleaning the fireplace.

9 Tunnels

Lie flat on back with knees bent and feet flat on floor. Hollow your back to make a tunnel, then press it firmly on the floor again. Repeat six times at least as this exercise helps posture.

10 Learning to relax

Lie on your left side, bend left leg slightly, and right one much more. Keep left arm lying near the spine and right one bent towards your face. Now . . . let all your muscles go . . . one by one. Close eyes lightly and repeat inwardly 'Relax . . . feet,' 'Relax . . . ankles' until every part of your body is more restful. Breathe gently and quietly. Practise this frequently, lying on floor or bed. Towards the end of pregnancy, this is the ideal position to ensure peaceful sleep. Many books will give other ideas for relaxation and peaceful Yoga positions which will help you to relax.

Other exercises help, too

If possible, try to have a good, brisk walk daily, or swim or cycle until about six months pregnant if you do this normally. Walking is the perfect exercise as it stimulates the circulation, prevents insomnia, aids the appetite and helps to keep your muscles firm.

Posture in pregnancy is most important. When sitting, ensure that your back is supported so that you avoid strain on muscles and joints. Never sit in a slouched position. It is far better to lie flat on a settee than slumped-up in an arm-chair. If you prefer an armchair, sit up fairly straight, but rest your feet on a low stool whenever possible. This helps to prevent varicose veins and relieves 'tired' feet.

When standing, keep your weight evenly between your heels and the balls of your feet, then tighten your buttocks and tummy muscles and stand 'tall'. Avoid standing for long periods when possible. Use a kitchen stool when preparing vegetables or washing dishes, and make some excuse not to stand chatting to every neighbour you meet when out shopping. Unnecessary standing aggravates piles, varicose veins and swollen feet.

Avoid lifting heavy weights when possible, but, if necessary, brace your abdomen, bend your knees, keep your back straight, then hold the weight close to you and lift it by straightening your knees. This enables the weight to be borne by the strong thigh and buttock muscles instead of by your over-burdened back.

Learn to sit, stand, lift and work in the positions of least strain for this will help you to avoid fatigue besides making your movements more graceful.

5 Ante-natal visits

Whether you attend your doctor or an ante-natal clinic during pregnancy, you will be expected to make a visit every four weeks until you are 28 weeks pregnant, every two weeks from then until you are 36 weeks pregnant then every week until you are confined. If any complication arises, or if you suffer from any disease such as diabetes, high blood pressure or heart trouble your doctor may want to see you more frequently.

Why are ante-natal visits necessary?

You may wonder why it is considered essential for you to visit a doctor regularly especially if you feel in excellent health as many women do during the waiting months. First, your doctor likes to know how you and the foetus inside you are progressing and how you are enjoying your pregnancy. He will be pleased to answer any questions you may ask on these occasions and will offer you his advice. By checking your condition at frequent intervals your doctor may be able to make your pregnancy more enjoyable and by noticing any unusual symptoms he may be able to prevent complications arising later in the pregnancy.

Watching the weight gain

Any woman who gains excessive weight during pregnancy runs the risk of developing the condition of pre-eclampsia. Most obstetricians consider that you should try not to gain more than 12.5 kg (28 lb) preferably rather less. Any extra poundage you gain during pregnancy is most difficult to lose after the birth.

Your weight gain will not be spread equally over the nine months. During the first 20 weeks a gain of 3.5 g (8 lbs) is about average, and about 14 to 20 lbs in the last half of pregnancy. During the last twenty weeks particularly your doctor will watch your weight carefully. Try not to gain more than 0.5 g (1 lb) per week during this period as any gain over 1 kg (2 lb) may indicate excess fat or fluid retention.

Checking your blood-pressure

At each ante-natal visit your blood-pressure will be taken and doctor will check that you have no swelling of the hands, face, feet or legs. Some slight swelling of the ankles is normal towards evening during pregnancy but swelling of the legs in the morning or of the hands and face at any time is a danger sign. Always report any swelling to your doctor, and any blurring of your vision or severe headache.

Doctor will test your urine at every visit for the presence of albumen (protein) which often reveals a pre-eclamptic condition. If any of these symptoms occur, follow your doctor's instructions implicitly for if they are neglected serious complications may arise. Your doctor may just suggest some restriction in your diet, such as avoiding salt and salty foods, and he may prescribe diuretic tablets to get rid of the extra water (and salt) which you have retained. When you are advised to rest at home, do not be tempted to ignore the suggestion because you feel well.

When the symptoms necessitate it, doctor will suggest rest in hospital where you will be given sedative drugs while the nurses and doctors can watch your blood pressure, weight gain, and the growth of the baby constantly.

Ante-natal classes

Many mothers-to-be enter labour in a tense, anxious state because they expect pain during childbirth through lack of knowledge of their own body and the birth processes. They may have a 'conditioned reflex' because of hearing exaggerated tales about painful labours experienced by other women. To avoid this, it is advisable to receive some instruction and practise certain exercises during pregnancy, so that you can approach the birth of your baby with confidence and joy.

Local authority ante-natal classes

Ante-natal classes are arranged for expectant mothers by most local authorities and maternity units. These include instruction in the elementary physiology of pregnancy, labour and lactation, and may include instruction in mothercraft. Some classes are devoted to exercises designed principally to teach you to relax during labour and especially during uterine contractions. They instruct you in the special breathing techniques that should be practised during the first and second stages of labour.

The National Childbirth Trust

This registered charity holds classes during the last three months of pregnancy and a modest fee is charged for the course. Eight two-hour classes include an explanation of pregnancy and labour, ante-natal and post-natal exercises, breathing and relaxation techniques helpful during labour, how father can help, feeding, caring and adjusting to the new baby, an informal discussion and a post-natal gathering.

6 Avoiding complications in pregnancy

Consitpation

Many women suffer from some degree of constipation occasionally during pregnancy. Every effort should be made to maintain a regular normal motion by eating roughage-containing foods such as wholewheat bread, muesli, bran, dates, prunes, raisins, salads, green vegetables and raw fruit. Drink two glasses of water on rising and some water between meals. Walking, exercises and housework help to prevent bowel stasis.

Miscarriage

A miscarriage is often nature's way of expelling an imperfect foetus. If a first baby is lost, it is important not to grieve unduly. Wait four months before trying to conceive again. When you have had one or two miscarriages previously, it is advisable to avoid intercourse during the normal period times. After this the foetus is more firmly fixed in the womb.

Always report any vaginal bleeding to your doctor immediately and lie down until he arrives. Sometimes a few days' complete rest can save the baby.

Varicose veins, vulval veins and haemorrhoids

When resting, either lie flat or with the feet raised on a stool. Avoid unnecessary standing. During a walk, do not be tempted to stand chatting to anyone you meet. Use a kitchen stool while washing dishes or clothes, preparing vegetables or ironing. Constipation aggravates these problems. Splashing cold water on distended veins or sore piles helps to tone up the areas.

Wear support tights or elastic stockings if varicose veins are painful or severe. Often they disappear after the baby's birth. Report any veins or piles to your doctor, especially when painful.

Swollen ankles and tired feet

Slight swelling of the ankles and heaviness in the feet often occur owing to the extra pressure from above, and may be worse by evening. Report to doctor and rest feet in a raised position when possible. Persevere with foot exercises to stimulate circulation in the legs.

Backache

This can prove troublesome during the last weeks. Keep an erect posture when walking or sitting. Do not wear high-heeled shoes which throw the body out of alignment. Sleep on a firm mattress. Gentle massage by husband may ease pain and relax tired lumbar muscles. A hot water bottle can prove a comfort.

Stretch marks

These are more likely to develop if you are overweight, having twins or carrying an excessive quantity of amniotic fluid. Some women like to apply a little olive oil, baby lotion or lanoline to the lower abdomen and breasts at night to keep the skin more elastic. Wearing a 'sleep' bra during the night during the final months may help to prevent stretch marks on breasts or sagging breasts after the birth.

Heartburn and indigestion

This is common during the last 12 weeks when the stomach is displaced by the enlarged uterus. Your doctor may prescribe an antacid medicine to relieve discomfort. Try sleeping with several pillows to keep your head raised. Avoid fatty and fried foods. If you drink fluid an hour before a meal and eat the food dry, this can relieve the discomfort.

Cramp and shooting pains

These may be due to calcium deficiency. Drink extra milk or eat more cheese. Your doctor may order a syrup containing calcium.

Dental decay

As your baby draws its calcium requirements from you, your teeth are more liable to decay during pregnancy. Dental treatment is free during pregnancy and for a year afterwards. Visit your dentist when your pregnancy is confirmed. Have any treatment recommended. Clean teeth regularly within ten minutes of eating any meal.

Mental changes

A husband should understand that you may suffer from mood changes for no apparent reason. Sometimes you will feel happier than ever before, while at other times you may feel depressed, irritable or over-emotional. Talk over any worries with your husband, as sympathetic understanding is consoling. You may be anxious in case pregnancy makes you unattractive to your husband but he will assure you it enhances his love for you.

Insomnia

Sleeplessness may be due to anxiety, an over-active baby or discomfort owing to your increasing size. Lying on your side in the 'relaxing' position with the upper leg placed well over the lower one will enable you to place the 'bump' actually on the mattress. Dreams may be due to hormonal changes. A warm (not hot) bath followed by drinking a glass of warm milk containing one tablespoonful of honey will often induce sleep. Once in bed practise the relaxation technique to ease bodily tensions.

Toxaemia of pregnancy

During your regular ante-natal visits to your doctor or clinic any rise in blood pressure, albumen in the urine or swollen ankles may indicate the beginning of toxaemia. Bed rest at home or in hospital may be essential. Sedatives and medicines will be ordered. Gaining excessive weight and eating too much salt appear to aggravate this serious trouble.

Breech presentation

Until the 30th week of pregnancy a baby moves around in the amniotic sac, then it tends to settle with its head over the mother's pelvis. When the doctor discovers a baby's buttocks are nearest to the cervix, he may try to turn the breech baby into a cephalic presentation with its head downwards. If a breech birth proves necessary, the mother need not worry as doctors and midwives are experienced in delivering these babies.

Morning sickness

If this has continued after the end of the third month your doctor will advise you about diet, obtaining extra rest and taking walks in the fresh air. Report any nausea or sickness during the later months.

Is love-making dangerous?

Many women experience an increased sexual desire during pregnancy. Normal marital relations can be enjoyed although after the fith or sixth month coitus will be more comfortable for the woman if she lies on her left side with her husband lying behind her. Some doctors advise refraining from inter-course during the last month in case the penile stimulation triggers off a premature delivery.

7 Requirements for Mum and the baby

Maternity clothes today are elegant and can be obtained in a wide variety of styles, from loose sleeveless dresses to T-shirts and slacks. Any woman who cannot visit suitable shops can obtain a free catalogue from Mothercare-by-Post, Cherry Tree Road, Watford, WD2 5SH, England, or from any Mothercare store. This attractively produced magazine lists all essential items for pregnant mums, babies and older children. It enables you to discover prices and types of various products without standing around in shops.

The enlarging breasts should be supported by a brassiere with a good uplift, wide shoulder straps and a wide band below the breasts.

Choose shoes with heels of moderate height and thickness to enable you to maintain balance and posture during pregnancy.

Maternity support tights provide support for the legs and help to prevent varicose veins. An adjustable waistband allows continued wear without constriction and supports the tummy without compression.

Requirements for baby

Choose a well-balanced pram of the right height and weight for you to push. A large pram may look attractive but requires considerable space in the hall. Many women prefer a light-weight pram with a folding chassis. It needs a firm mattress with waterproof cover and an attachable canopy. No pillow is required until baby is old enough to be propped up. You need four small sheets, two blankets and two pram covers. A pillow-case makes an excellent mattress cover. A carry-cot on secure stand is ideal for the first three months, or use a large padded drawer. Firm mattress (with waterproof cover), four to six flannelette sheets, three cellular wool blankets. No pillow.

Baby bath with firm base. Changing table, or chest of drawers to hold baby's clothes. Top proves useful when changing or 'topping and tailing' baby.

Low nursing chair. Baby basket containing toilet articles, safety pins, etc.

Two bath towels. Towelling apron for your own use.

Screen to protect baby from draughts can be made from a clothes-maiden. Useful, too, for holding towels, clothes, etc.

Even if you intend breast-feeding baby, buy two bottles and teats for use when giving baby fruit juice, water, or expressed breast milk. If bottle-feeding baby, buy six bottles and six teats so that a day's feeds can be prepared at once, then placed in the refrigerator.

Choose plastic, wide-necked bottles. Bottle brush. Sterilising container and sterilising chemicals in powder or liquid form.

Two enamel buckets . . . one for soiled and one for wet napkins.

Some form of heating is necessary in the nursery during winter.

Layette for baby

Buy second-size clothes as babies grow quickly. Three vests with envelope shoulders, three nightdresses — no waistband, or three to four stretch suits, three cardigans with button fastenings (not ribbons).

Woollen caps, mitts and socks for a winter baby.

Two cellular woollen shawls or blankets for carrying baby.

Two sleeping bags for a winter baby.

Four pairs of plastic pants (legs must be loose enough to allow ventilation).

Two dozen Turkish towelling napkins and one dozen muslin ones as liners. If you intend to use disposable napkins, buy a few towelling ones for emergencies. Disposables are excellent for first few weeks when you are tied or when travelling with baby. Nappy liners. One pram suit. Do not buy dresses etc. for babies often receive clothes as gifts.

Hydroscopic napkins are useful as urine passes through, leaving baby's skin dry.

Requirements for hospital

For Mum . . . three nighties with front opening, dressing-gown, slippers, three nursing bras (front opening), two pairs briefs, two sanitary belts, one packet maternity sanitary pads, toilet articles, cosmetics, writing materials, stamps, books or magazines, knitting, sugar (if taken in drinks). Bottle of fruit squash. Two towels.

For baby . . . a full set of clothes for taking baby home. Toilet articles, two towels, safety pins. Ask at your hospital if they provide a list, as hospitals' needs vary.

Be prepared in good time

In case baby should arrive prematurely, have your case packed during the seventh month.

Breast-feeding or bottle-feeding?

Breast-feeding is a baby's birthright. No-one has ever improved on a mother's milk for her baby. This method is the easiest, cheapest and quickest way to feed a baby, while it provides the infant with some resistance to disease. A woman benefits from breast-feeding in two ways: the sucking action encourages the womb to return to normal quickly, while mother and child achieve a closeness and understanding through physical contact.

Preparing the breasts

Wash breasts daily then sponge with cold water to firm the tissues. If nipples are small, pull them out daily, roll gently between fingers using a little lanoline or cold cream. Drink at least one pint of milk daily with water between meals. From the 30th week, the breasts should be 'expressed' by placing both hands round the breast and pressing gently towards the nipple. Some yellow secretion will appear and this treatment helps to keep the ducts of the breasts open and encourages an ample supply of milk later.

Bottle-feeding

If you decide to bottle-feed your baby, your breasts require no treatment although you should wear the supporting brassieres until after baby's birth.

Modern milk mixtures are of high quality. A breast-feeding mother requires a considerable amount of rest daily, so if you cannot manage plenty of rest periods it is better to choose a suitable baby feeding formula.

Equipment for bottle-feeding baby

Six feeding bottles (choose ones with wide necks which are easy to clean)
Eight teats (some bottles have special teats)
a graduated glass measuring jug
Three or four teat covers (if teats cannot be reversed)
Large plastic measuring spoon (metal is affected by sterilising liquid)
Two small plastic spoons (for giving cod liver oil, orange juice or medicine)
Two bottle brushes (to be kept in a jar of detergent solution)
An electric bottle-warmer is useful
Sterilising tank to hold all equipment (or two small ones)
Pot containing salt for cleaning teats
Sterilising lotion (obtainable in liquid, tablet or powder form)
This list provides for you to make all the day's feeds at once if you have a refrigerator for storage.

Your maternity benefits

Maternity benefits are available to you under the National Health Insurance Scheme. For full details of these obtain forms N1 17A, BM4 and M11 from your local social security office or maternity or child health clinic.

The maternity grant is a lump sum payment to help you with the general expenses of labour and is paid on either your own or your husband's national insurance contributions (but not on both). You may claim the grant at any time from fourteen weeks before your baby is expected up to three months after the birth. If you claim later you may lose the grant unless you have a good reason for the delay. The grant cannot be paid at all if you submit your claim more than a year after your confinement.

If you have twins, triplets, etc the maternity grant is paid for each child who lives more than twelve hours. It is paid even if your child is stillborn as long as pregnancy lasted twenty-eight weeks.

Check to find if you need to pay any outstanding contributions for any paid after your baby is born will not count towards the grant.

If you are single you can claim only on the basis of your own insurance contributions.

If you are a widow expecting your late husband's baby you can claim on his contributions or your own.

If you are divorced you can claim the grant only on your own contributions unless you claim it before you have the baby and you were married to the man on whose contribution card you are claiming for any part of the period starting eleven weeks before, and ending with, the date of your confinement.

Maternity allowance

If you have been working and paying full insurance contributions you are also entitled to a maternity allowance whether you are married or single. This allowance is provided to make it easier for you to give up work in reasonable time before the birth, in the interests of both you and your baby.

This allowance should be claimed by completing Form BM4 between the fourteenth and eleventh weeks before your baby is expected, even though you may continue working for a while after the fourteenth week. If you claim after the eleventh week before the expected date of birth you may lose the allowance for the weeks before you claim.

If you meet the contribution conditions the allowance is paid weekly by a book of orders which you can cash at the Post Office. If your baby arrives late inform the local Social Security office and enclose the baby's birth certificate or the certificate of confinement supplied by your doctor or midwife. The allowance is paid for eighteen weeks, beginning eleven weeks before the expected date of confinement but not for any time when paid work is done.

Other benefits

If your income is low you can obtain free milk and vitamins by completing form M11. You will be exempt from prescription charges while pregnant and for the year following baby's birth. Free family planning is available for anyone from N.H.S. family planning clinics or for women from most N.H.S. doctors.

You are entitled to free dental treatment during pregnancy and for the year after baby is born. It is advisable to have a dental check-up immediately pregnancy is confirmed. You can find details in leaflet M11 from Post Offices and Social Security Offices.

8 When baby arrives

By the thirty-sixth week your baby is almost fully mature and his body and limbs are becoming rounder and plumper. His body is covered with a barrier cream called vernix which protects the skin from abrasions and from hardening. If he is born prematurely now he stands more than ninety per cent chance of survival.

Approach of labour

With a first confinement baby's head usually enters the pelvis about two to four weeks before labour starts. After baby has 'dropped' you will find the enlargement of the upper part of your abdomen is less noticeable.

The first indication of labour is that you become conscious of contractions of the womb occurring at intervals of half an hour or more, often accompanied by a low backache. If these become irregular and then disappear this may be a 'false' labour. Do not feel embarrassed if you go to hospital then discover it was a false alarm as it is sometimes difficult to differentiate.

Most babies arrive during the fortieth week though they can come a week or more before or after the estimated date of delivery. Sometimes the first indication that baby is due to be born is a mood change. One woman says: 'I felt like spring-cleaning the house' while another declares: 'Suddenly all my tiredness left me and I tacked all the family washing.'

Onset of true labour

The first sign may be the loss of the plug of sticky blood-stained mucus which had sealed the neck of the womb. Warn the hospital or midwife if you have this 'show', or if you have a gushing of liquid from the vagina, or when your contractions are coming regularly every 10 or 15 minutes.

The uterus has several groups of muscles which become enlarged during pregnancy. Some stretch from one side of the cervix, go over the top of the uterus and down to the other side of the cervix. These have to contract to pull up the cervix to create the opening for baby's birth. Other muscles which encircle the cervix have to relax during labour to allow the cervix to rise up.

Once you enter hospital remember you are in the care of experts so try to relax. The pubic hair is usually shaved for cleanliness and to prevent infection, your urine is tested, blood pressure taken and a midwife or doctor will examine you to find out how much the cervix has dilated.

If you experience the 'breaking of the waters' while at home it is important to reach hospital quickly. The membranes which form the amniotic sac around the baby have ruptured, which means labour may occur within a few hours.

You will have been told at the ante-natal classes about the procedure in hospital, and the three stages of labour. During the first and longest stage, the cervix has to be drawn up and the birth canal widened, during the second stage your baby is born, while the placenta is expelled in the final stage.

The first stage of labour

You will be encouraged to walk about, read or watch television until the contractions become uncomfortably strong, when you will feel happier relaxing in bed. You will be given a pain-relieving drug, sedative or analgesic when this is necessary. You can help yourself to speed up labour by practising the relaxation and breathing exercises you have learned during your pregnancy. Breathe slowly and deeply through each contraction. By being prepared, relaxed and unafraid you keep tension at bay.

If your husband has attended some of the preparation classes with you and can be with you during this stage of labour, he will reassure you and remind you of the breathing and muscular control techniques.

By co-operating with your midwife or doctor, you will feel more comfortable. In many cases, labour is controlled to some extent. By the use of a drug which stimulates the contractions of the uterus, labour can often be shortened considerably.

Episiotomy

Many doctors perform an episiotomy, which is merely making a tiny cut in the perineum so that the vaginal opening is large enough to enable baby's head to pass through without tearing the tissues. This cut is painless as a local anaesthetic is injected first, then it can be stitched up neatly afterwards and heals quickly.

The second stage in labour

Towards the start of the second stage contractions may be coming every two minutes and last for a minute or so. Do not push down yet until the dilation of the cervix is complete, then the midwife will tell you: 'When the next contraction comes, take a deep breath and bear down.' If the bag of waters is still intact, it will rupture at this stage.

You may feel pressure on the anus with a sensation of wanting to open the bowels. During this stage you will be comfortably propped up on two or three pillows while you grasp your legs behind the thighs and pull upwards during contractions. Relax as much as possible during the 'rest' periods as this stage requires a tremendous amount of energy.

Delivery of the baby

For the actual birth of your baby you may be advised to lie on your back with knees bent and legs widely separated, or lying on your left side with an attendant holding the right leg upwards.

During the 'crowning' of baby's head (when it reaches the exit) you will be told to stop bearing down and to breathe in and out rapidly. This panting enables the midwife or doctor to deliver the head slowly and gently to prevent lacerations. It is an exciting moment when you see your baby's head appear. Do not be amazed if someone says: 'You've got a ginger (or black) haired baby' if neither you nor your husband have hair this colour, for a baby's hair alters in colour within a few weeks. The body slides out within a couple of minutes during the next uterine contraction. His first cry is like music to your ears.

Baby's treatment at birth

The umbilical cord is clamped and cut about 5.1 cm (2 ins) away from the navel. He may be held upside down for a moment and his nose and mouth may be gently sucked out by the midwife using a mucus extractor. She will wrap him up warmly and place him in your arms for a short time. At last you know if your long-awaited child is a boy or a girl. If your husband is present he will be proud of the physcial efforts you have made and of the child you have both produced. Probably he will say: 'What a wonderful experience to see our baby born.'

The third stage of labour

Once baby has arrived, all that remains is for the expulsion of the placenta, membranes and cord. This may take up to 20 minutes, but is virtually painless. You may be asked to push slightly to help the midwife deliver them. If you require stitches these will be inserted then you will have a wash-down and a drink, or food too, if hungry, before settling down for a sleep. Feeling your tummy flat again is another pleasant experience.

Your stay in hospital

If you have decided to breast feed your baby the midwife will help to get feeding established. For about three days a fluid called colostrum is produced by the breasts.

About the third day the breasts tend to become rather engorged as milk arrives but this will disappear as baby's sucking becomes stronger.

You will be given some medicine or tablets to dry up the unwanted liquid if you intend to bottle-feed your baby, and fluids may be restricted for a day or two.

Although you will be allowed out of bed within 24 hours of baby's birth, remember you need plenty of rest after the physical and emotional effort of childbirth. Many mothers are transferred home within 48 hours if baby is thriving and they have adequate help in the home. Members of the Community Nursing Service will visit you at home and advise you about caring for baby and check on your health.

A paediatric doctor will examine your baby thoroughly before your discharge to exclude any abnormality. Most babies are born perfect, but if any treatment is necessary it can be started as early as possible.

You will be given a date when to attend the hospital for a post-natal check-up in six weeks' time and this should not be missed. The midwife or physiotherapist will also remind you of the importance of practising your post-natal exercises daily.

Most new mothers suffer from an attack of 'the blues' about the third day after the birth, but this is simply a reaction after your months of pregnancy and the birth. Usually this clears up within a few hours and you can start to look forward to a happy family life.